WEIGHT LOSS

The only guide you will ever need

BRADLEY CONNER

Table of Contents

Who is this book for?

There are no pre-requisites for this book. It assumes no prior knowledge of nutrition or exercise sciences. That being said, if you are expecting to lose 20 pounds in a month, from this book then you would be disappointed. However, if you want to get healthier again, lose excess weight and keep it off for the rest of your life than you should read this book. If you want to keep metabolic disorders like diabetes, hypertension, heart disease, dementia, cancer at bay then you should read this book. There are no strict diets, no hardcore exercise plans and weight loss programs in this book. This book merely contains some fundamental and very simple principles that, if followed, can keep you healthy. Even if you are not trying to lose weight, I would recommend to go through this book at least once, you may find some useful gems.

Finally, I would like to emphasize that the purpose of this book is not to give you an ultimate diet or weight loss program but to question the efficacy of such programs that are sold and marketed to us. It is ok to ask questions and it is ok to have doubts. Einstein once said that "The greater the doubt the greater the awakening".

How to read this book

This book contains 16 simple habits in decreasing order of priority to help you achieve a better health. The first two principles, in my opinion are the most important. I've categorized the habits into three sections: critically important (1 and 2); very important (3 to 5) and important (6 to 16). If you have a BMI of over 30. I would recommend to start with the first 2 habits for 2 weeks and then incorporate 3 through 5. You can live a very healthy life if you follow only the first 5 habits. The remaining (6 through 16) are addendums to the top 5 and would help you achieve your health goals faster and would help you stay healthy.
Here is a brief description of the top 5.

1. **Stay away from processed food**: This section covers the implications of consuming highly processed food on our health and why it is much better to give up on processed food.
2. **Keep a Journal**: If you are serious about your goals whether the goals are related to health, weight loss, finance or career, it is important to keep track of your progress. Without a journal it's like wandering around aimlessly because your GPS is broken. You can vision what your destination looks like but you'll spend an awful lot of time and efforts to get there, if at all.
3. **Eat more fiber from plants, vegetables and whole grains:** Fiber plays a key role in regulating the absorption of glucose in small intestine, health of our microbiome, fullness and satiety and mitigation of chronic metabolic disorders.
4. **Sugar control:** This section covers a few important facts about America's ever-increasing appetite for sugar and how sugar is as addictive as some of the drugs, if not more.
5. **Exercise:** Exercise is the single most useful thing one can do to improve health, well-being and longevity but it is almost useless when it comes to short term weight loss. Therefore, it is often ignored by people following fad diets for quick weight loss leading to reduction in metabolic rate, eating disorders and hormonal imbalances.

Introduction

A few months ago, I saw a presentation by Dr. Robert Lustig in which he mentioned about an article published in the Atlantic in 2014 by Zeke Emmanuel. Zeke Emmanuel, Rahm Emmanuel's brother, is an oncologist at the University of Pennsylvania and the architect of Obamacare. The article is called "Why I hope to die at 75" because he wanted to justify how Obamacare was going to work. In the article he said that the current generation of Americans will probably live longer than the previous generation, but they are likely to be sick and incapacitated. Zeke then raised the question: Is it worth living beyond 75 if you are crippled and suffering from a chronic illness. More than 50 percent of the health care cost spent in this country is in the last month of life and that's why his argument was that we don't need health care after 75. As logical as it may sound, it is preposterous.

In the entire Affordable Care Act, which is nearly 1000 pages long, the word "diet" is not mentioned. Weight loss and exercise are mentioned but diet is not mentioned. President Obama promised that we could put 32 million sick people onto the rolls and we would pay for this by providing preventative services. The argument was that by providing healthcare access to everyone (so that everyone could see their doctors), we could keep people out of the emergency room. However, after Obamacare was instituted there was an uptick in ER visits not a downturn. And because insurance companies were capped to make profit, three of the big insurers Aetna, United and Humana left the exchanges. In fact, under Obamacare the cost for diabetes went from 245 billion to 345 billion. Does that sound very preventative? And under Trump-care we have Mick Mulvaney, Trump's budget director saying, you brought this upon yourself so" no health care for you" which is even more preposterous.

The problem is Obamacare, Trump-care and every other care ignores two very embarrassing truths. First, there is no medicalized prevention for chronic metabolic diseases. There are no medicines that can fix the disorder, there is just long-term treatment. A meta-analysis of type-2 diabetes prevention strategies looked into various lifestyle and drugs and their impact on the patient. What they observed is that both lifestyle changes and drugs have statistically significant impact on mitigating the impact of the metabolic syndrome on the body. However, the number needed to treat (NNT) diabetes using these drugs and medical procedures is 25. That means, you have to institute preventative strategies on 25 people to prevent diabetes in one. Considering we have a 9.4 percent diabetes prevalence right now and a 40 percent pre-diabetes prevalence we would have to basically treat half the population and we won't even get anything out of it at twenty-five to one. The second inconvenient truth is that you can't fix health care until you fix health and you can't fix health until you fix diet and you can't fix diet until you fix processed food!

Stop eating processed food, start cooking

Processed food diet can be defined as a diet that is high in processed meat or sugar, low in fiber with very little ingredients in their natural form and enhanced with fillers and chemical additives to make the food last long and taste good.

Facts:
1. Usually the food is processed to achieve the following things 1) high shelf life 2) low ingredient cost 3) better taste 4) make the consumers ask for more for better and consistent cash flow 5) adding external micronutrients to make the food look appealing nutritionally (which can be very deceiving)
2. Processing the food removes fibers, omega-3's, anti-oxidants and practically all micronutrients. Since the nutritional value of this type of food is so low, pests and microbes don't consume it and that's why the shelf life is more. In natural unprocessed food like fruits, vegetables, dairy and meat the decay rate is very high since they are highly nutritious. Thus, processing makes the food so devoid of nutrients that even pests don't want to eat it. However, with the addition of sugar, salt, saturated fats and other additives the food can be made palatable for humans. And not only just palatable, meta-analysis suggests that food companies spend a substantial amount of their budget researching chemicals that can make the nutritionally devoid but calorie dense food appealing to us. To such an extent that some of us are addicted to it.
3. In the past 30 years the rate of obesity and major metabolic disorders like diabetes, heart diseases, cancer, dementia have reached epidemic proportions. In the late 1970's we falsely convicted fats in our diet as the major perpetrator of obesity and decreased our dietary fat intake. The food industry, in order to keep the food palatable and to keep the cash flow going decided to substitute fat with sugar, sugar substitutes and other additives. Sugar, it turns out is highly addictive and much worse than the fats it replaced. In fact, removal of fats especially unsaturated fats made the situation worse worldwide. According to CDC the obesity among Americans, has increased by 250% over the last 30 years and diabetes has increased by over 400%.
4. Some of the characteristics of processed food are: 1) They are cheap. 2) They can be produced very quickly. 3) They are available everywhere. 4) They have a long list of ingredients and often esoteric ingredients which you and I haven't heard of. 5) 75% of all processed food in the supermarket contain added sugar or sugar substitutes (even foods like bread, pasta, ketchup and chips) 6) They may contain synthetically added micronutrients or fiber or BCAA's (Branched Chain Amino Acids) to make them look nutritionally appealing. 7) They taste very good, addictively good! 8) They are served in pretty large containers. In fact, their meal size or serving size has increased substantially over the last few years.
5. The food companies invest a huge amount of money in market, advertising and sales of processed food. Even their location in the supermarket aisles is chosen to increase sales (products placed at eye level in the aisles have been shown to sell more). Interestingly, natural foods like fruits, vegetables, whole grains, even dairy, fish and meat don't require any marketing or slogans or bloated advertisements touting how healthy they are.
6. There is overwhelming empirical and experimental research evidence to suggest that switching from processed food to natural or very lightly processed food changes our microbiome within our bodies, increase hormone profile, could trigger leptin response essential in insulin regulation and would make us feel less hungry when insulin is not running amok in our system.

Recommendations:

1. This book contains a lot of advice on food, exercise and health. However, if there is one advice which trumps all of the others is this: Stop eating processed food, eat real food, start cooking. If you follow this advice all the others would work, if you don't, it would be very hard if not impossible to make the others work in the long term. (Yes, there would be occasional bouts of success here and there but if you revert back to processed food it's very likely that you'll eventually undo all your achievements). Also, please avoid sugary beverages and soda as much as possible and try to replace them with water. We'll go through this in more detail in the section on Water.
2. I understand that most people today don't have the time for cooking but at least you can limit your intake of processed food and start eating more fruits and vegetables.
3. For those who don't know how to cook, cooking is actually not that hard. You only need some very basic ingredients to start cooking and once you get a hang of it you might actually enjoy it. Personally, in our house, we always keep these basic ingredients at home and we can make an excellent healthy meal with these in under 15 mins: Olive oil, vinegar, lemon, salt, (frozen) spinach, onion, tomato, salmon or tuna, black beans.
4. There is an excellent course on Coursera.org by Dr. Maya Adam called "Stanford Introduction to Food and Health", in which the topic of cooking and processed food has been covered extensively. If you want to learn more about it, I would highly recommend watching the course videos. It's available for free.

Interesting Fact: The Medium soda cup size at McDonalds's in USA is at 21oz whereas the large cup size in Japan is at 20oz. The large cup size in US is 1.5 times the large cup size in Japan.

Keep a Journal

Learning how to journal is not just about recording parameters like weight, calories consumed, type of meal, numbers of sets and reps, etc.; but it's also about writing about your goals, vision, your thoughts in that moment, what went right and what went wrong, what did you anticipate and what really happened and finally, what you plan to do in future. Writing a journal has three major advantages: a) it slows down time such that you are not in a hurry. You can think rationally without stress. As you probably know stress increases cortisol which impedes the Prefrontal Cortex function. b) Our past experience is a huge treasure chest of ideas and knowledge. Even failure in the past can be a great mentor and we could learn from it provided it is properly documented. c) It's a great habit to document your daily life and it only requires about 10 minutes. It's often said that success is not one great moment but a series of good habits repeated daily.

Facts:
1. Research suggests that people who keep a track of their daily goals are more likely to achieve them.
2. Our mind goes through over 5000 different thoughts every day. For most of us, it is often very hard to focus amidst the clutter of daily life. No wonder so many of us are suffering from ADD. Research suggests that only 2.5% of the population is capable of multi-tasking without getting a surge of cortisol. So where does writing a journal fit in all this? Decision fatigue is a serious problem and it can cause a lot of anxiety and stress. As mentioned before writing down thoughts, action plans not only declutter the mind but help us anticipate and avoid future problems. People who keep a daily journal are more focused, more responsible and keep themselves accountable.
3. Patients who aspired to improve their health but stopped recording their parameters like body weight, food intake, sleep, food experiences etc., were 15 times more likely to not only not achieve their objectives but undo whatever health goals they have already achieved.
4. If you have goals, the purpose of a daily journal is to keep you on track and not to lose sight of them in the hustle and chaos of daily life.

Recommendations:

1. Spend at least 10 mins jotting down your weight, sleep quality and how you feel early in the morning when you get up.
2. Keep track of your food and meal parameters like: a) what did you eat b) was it heavily processed (check the definition of processed food diet in section 1) or cooked at home c) water consumption d) number of calories and e) how much of vegetables, fruits and whole grain food did you consume in this meal? (We'll go through all these parameters in the later section)
3. If possible provide as much details as you can. It might feel like a chore right now but if you practice you might actually enjoy monitoring your progress. More importantly, the details might seem redundant right now but they usually turn out to be priceless in future.

What's so special about fiber?

Fiber is considered one of the NUTRIENTS OF CONCERN for Americans according to the Dietary Guidelines for Americans. We, on an average consume only about 47% of the recommended dietary fiber. More than 90% of us do not maintain the daily food intake of fruits and vegetables based on the federal fruits and vegetables intake recommendations.

Facts:

1. Research suggests that dietary fiber plays a key role in weight control, mitigating the risk of diabetes and other metabolic disorders. When you eat food high in sugar but devoid of fiber, it is quickly absorbed leading to a huge spike in glucose and insulin. However, fiber both soluble and insoluble slows down the absorption of glucose in the small intestine leading to a gradual spike in insulin.
2. There are 5 types of fiber sources: Fruits, vegetables, whole grains, seeds and beans/legumes. According to the FDA an average adult needs 28 to 40g of fiber in their diet every day. There are two kinds of fiber: soluble and insoluble fiber. Insoluble fiber moves through the large intestine and is disposed-off whereas soluble fiber helps prevent blood glucose and insulin spikes by slowing down the absorption of nutrients in the small intestine. It makes us feel fuller and therefore we are less prone to overeating when we eat food containing lots of fiber. Nuts, seeds, lentils are some of the common sources of soluble fiber.
3. There is another classification of fiber based on the origin: dietary fiber and functional fiber. All the fiber we obtain from food in its natural form is called dietary fiber. The fiber which is artificially added to processed food to increase its fiber content is called functional fiber.
4. Research suggest that our microbiome (aka gut bacteria) feed on the soluble component of the fiber and release compounds which are anti-inflammatory. Dietary fiber from whole foods, fruits and vegetables is the best fuel for our microbiome. Gut bacteria break down the soluble component of the fiber and other nutrients to produce short chain fatty acids which strengthen the immune system, produce anti-inflammatory compounds, improve the gut barrier and prevent the risk of cancer by reducing inflammation. The more fiber we eat from the plants, the more of these microbiomes inhabit our gut. The more diverse these microbiome species are, the healthier and more resilient our immune system becomes. However, eating processed food or food low in fiber changes the profile of our microbiome to such an extent that the species of healthy microbiome which regulate the gut barrier are significantly reduced in concentration and are often replaced by different species of gut bacteria. An imbalance in the species of "good" and "bad" bacteria can lead to deficient immune system, digestive problems and myriad of other disorders. There is significant empirical evidence based on mice studies that suggests that the microbiome species in obese mice are very different from those in healthy mice. Simply fixing our diet can improve the quality of our microbiome.
5. As an example, almonds contain a lot of calories, however, fiber prevents the absorption of some of those calories in upper intestine and keeps the blood sugar from rising which keeps the insulin down. Lower insulin level, keeps the liver safe and prevents weight gain. The fiber delivers more calories down the intestine so the bacteria end up chewing them instead of you absorbing them. Only about 80% (This number varies and is debatable based on latest research) of those calories are available for you to absorb.
6. Apart from fiber, fruits and vegetables provide numerous anti-oxidants and micronutrients. It has been observed that due to our increased dependence on processed food our intake of vegetables has decreased substantially over the last 30 years. Vegetables contain anti-oxidants which have been shown to mitigate angiogenesis and prevent cancer growth. In fact, depending on the type of cancer, anti-oxidants in certain fruits and vegetables are as potent as cancer drugs if not more. For more details on angiogenesis check out the Ted Talk by Dr William Li titled "Can we eat to starve cancer".

Recommendations:

1. The general rule of thumb is: at least 50% of your calories should come from unprocessed or lightly processed or home cooked plant sources.
2. Try to get diversity in fruits and vegetables.
3. If you have to get frozen or canned fruits and veggies from the supermarket please keep an eye on the sugar and especially salt content "per serving".
4. Document your daily fiber intake in your journal.

Sugar

Over the last 30 years our sugar consumption has increased dramatically leading to an exponential increase in serious metabolic disorders like diabetes, chronic heart disease, hypertension, dementia etc. Statistical analysis of processed food data suggests that majority of our sugar consumption comes from highly processed food and sugary beverages.

Facts:

1. Researchers conducted a study on mice where a group of mice were given cocaine for 4 days via a lever whenever the mice pressed the lever. After ensuring that the mice were addicted to cocaine, sugar was introduced on the 5th day. By the end of the 15th day all mice had stopped pressing the lever for cocaine altogether and were pressing the lever that delivered sugar at an average 40% higher frequency than on the 5th day.

2. In order to maintain a healthy body weight, people need to reduce their sugar intake especially from processed food. However, sugar is added to 75% of all processed food, even those that are not supposed to be sweet like sauces, ketchups, chips, condiments, breads etc.

3. One can of diet soda contains about 150 calories. It was observed that if the average food take of Americans were to go up by 150 calories the diabetes rate would go up by only 0.1%. However, if all those 150 calories are coming from sugar the diabetes rate would be go up 11 times i.e. by 1.1%. We are taking a lot more sugar than we were 30 years ago and we are getting addicted to sugar. Our insulin levels are on an average 3 times higher than what they used to be 3 decades ago. Another research concluded that one can of diet soda per day increases the risk of diabetes by 29%.

4. When sugar from processed food reaches the small intestine, it is quickly absorbed resulting in a quick spike in blood glucose level and insulin. Leptin, often called an energy expenditure hormone, is triggered by our adipose cells (fat), signaling the brain that we have enough energy reserves and we are no longer hungry. If the insulin level is too high, leptin signals to the hypothalamus are hindered. When insulin is running rampant in the system, it overwhelms cell mitochondria causing liver fat accumulation. However, even though there is fat accumulation we feel tired since our blood glucose level is low and we feel hungry since leptin signals to the hypothalamus are too week. Thus, we are getting fat due to too much sugar in our diet, while simultaneously feeling tired and hungry at the same time.

5. Sugar substitutes like corn syrup are used heavily in processed foods. Corn in its natural form when consumed doesn't lead to blood glucose and insulin spikes because it contains a lot of fiber and as discussed earlier, fiber slows down the absorption of sugar. However, when it is processed to produce high fructose corn syrup, fiber is removed.

6. According to World Health Organization's sugar intake guidelines, adults should restrict their sugar intake to less than 10% of the total daily caloric intake. The sugar intake for children should be reduced to 5%. However, these recommendations are applicable only for processed food focusing on sugar that is artificially added by manufacturers to increase their shelf life and make them more appealing to the customers. There recommendations do not apply to sugar in unprocessed/natural food like fruits, vegetables and nuts.

Recommendations:

1. Try to reduce the consumption of highly processed food, fast food and sugary beverages. In fact, you should completely eliminate sugary beverages and replace them with water or green tea.
2. As discussed in section 2 on journal and documentation. Introduce a column in your journal where you keep track of your daily sugar intake based on WHO guidelines. That means sugar, except those naturally found in fruits, vegetables and whole grains must be considered "added sugar" (including dairy). For example, if you ate 2 servings of cereal with 12g grams of added sugar per serving, one serving of Greek yogurt with 15g of added sugar and an apple, your total added sugar intake in that meal is 39 grams. Based on WHO guidelines you should limit your added sugar intake to 25 grams per day.

Exercise and Weight training

It is universally agreed among all health and fitness researches that working out regularly is the single best way for achieving good health, happiness and longevity. Physical activity or exercise constitutes 10 to 40 percent of our energy expenditure. Conversely, research suggest that exercise is not very useful for short term weight loss goals. Weight training however, will increase your metabolism and would lead to weight loss due to increased metabolic rate. Recent scientific publications also indicate that exercise is responsible for cognition and brain cell regeneration.

Facts:

1. Exercise and physical activity have a profound effect on our mood and is one of best ways to alleviate depression. (Several studies also provide conclusive evidence that helping others in need increases serotonin level which dramatically alleviates depression). After an intense workout our body releases endorphins which reduce the intensity of pain in our pain receptors, often resulting in a "euphoric" felling, also called a "runner's high". Endorphins therefore, increase a feeling of well-being and act as an analgesic similar to morphine, that's why people who work out regularly enjoy the feeling so much so that it's almost like an addiction to them. But it's not an addiction because unlike dopamine, endorphins mask the pain but if you overdo your workout you can substantially break down your tissues and extend the recovery time.
2. The benefits of exercise, weight training and physical activity are immense. I cannot go into each and every one of them here but here is a compendium of the documented benefits of exercise: a) increase in brain performance and memory b) increase in metabolism especially due to weight training c) reversal in metabolic disorders and fatty acid disease d) diabetes control e) cancer prevention f) better sex life g) can reverse aging h) has been shown to reduce stress i) better quality of sleep.
3. For weight loss the primary goal of exercise should not be losing calories but increasing metabolism by creating new muscle. More muscle hypertrophy means more metabolism in the long run. Although losing calories is important for weight loss, physical activity is a very small part of the total number of calories burnt by our bodies. The majority of the calories we eat are utilized by our body to run the vital organs and perform other critical functions. This is called the metabolism. Metabolism is very complex to estimate theoretically and can be dependent on several variables. In the laboratory it is measured by a calorimeter.

Recommendations:

1. If you haven't worked out in a long time, I would recommend starting out with some basic movements. You can start with the following 5 fundamental movements: Squat, deadlifts, farmer's walk, pull ups and push-ups. If you don't have a gym membership or don't have the time you can easily do these exercises at home. (The deadlifts, to start with, can be done using dumbbells). All these exercises are called "compound movements" and should form the backbone of your workout routine.
2. The lower body contains some of the biggest muscle groups in the body like glutes, hamstrings and quads. Stimulating them would lead to greater muscle fatigue/soreness, increase in metabolism and therefore more weight loss in the long term.
3. At the end of the day you can create a workout schedule any way you like and I am not going to give you any strict rules or strategies as to what is the most effective way to lose weight or to get ripped. All I am asking you to do is to focus on compound movements and work out EVERYDAY. You don't have to work out to the max every single day and you can do some lighter movement if you are sore but you should try and develop the habit of exercising every day. I've noticed that most of my clients who consider exercise as a chore, eventually give up. Research suggests that people who are discipline enough to do a difficult task every day for 90 days without interruption eventually develop the habit and retain the habit for a long time. (I would recommend: Meg Robbins book "5 second rule" and Jocko Willink's book "Extreme Ownership", if you are struggling to meet your goals due to lack of discipline)
4. Checkout Mark Rippetoe's videos on Back Squats, deadlifts, power cleans, "the press", etc. on YouTube. Those are some of the best "how to" exercise videos you'll find and they are all free.
5. Document your daily workout in your journal.

More Protein?

Apart from metabolism and physical work, the third component which is responsible for energy expenditure in our bodies is the Thermic effect of food. Our bodies expend energy to digest food and the amount of energy spent depends on the type of food. Usually fats require the lowest amount of energy to digest, approximately 5% of the total calorific values. Carbohydrates depending on the type of carbohydrate may require anywhere from 5 to 12%. Proteins however, have the highest thermic effect. The body expends anywhere from 20 to 30% of energy to digest protein. Doesn't that imply that we should eat more protein? Well, it depends!

Facts:

1. There are 9 essential amino acids that the body cannot produce on its own. They along with their substrates perform a wide variety of functions in our body and are quintessential to a healthy life. Deficiency in essential proteins could seriously compromise one or several systems in our body.
2. Protein along with fiber, also have a high satiety effect. Research has shown that people who eat more protein with fiber are less likely to overeat.
3. However, research also suggests that excessive consumption of animal protein especially red meat and processed meat can have long term negative effects on the body. That being said since very few plant-based proteins are complete proteins it is recommended to eat diverse plant sources to provide the body with all the essential amino acids it needs. For example: nuts, legumes, seeds and vegetables together in a single meal provide all the essential amino acids even though individually they are deficient in some.
4. There is an essential amino acid called L-methionine which is rare in plant-based sources and high in animal and dairy products like eggs, beef, chicken, etc. Methionine plays a very important part in the formation of cysteine, glutathione and angiogenesis. Angiogenesis is the process by which new blood vessels are formed from existing ones. Although angiogenesis plays a key role in growth and development, it is also responsible for cancer. Research on cancer suggest that there are several anti-angiogenesis compounds naturally present in fruits and vegetables which inhibit the growth of cancer. That's why eating highly processed animal protein coupled with empty calories devoid of any significant nutritional value is very unhealthy.
5. Consumption of food containing large amount of branched-chain amino acids (leucine, isoleucine and valine) can have deleterious effect on our health. Statistical analysis of obesity and BCAA data suggests that obese and insulin resistant individuals have higher levels of BCAAs. According to Dr. Robert Lustig high amounts of BCAAs are found in processed meat. There is a positive co-relation between BCAA concentration in blood and diabetes. In a research paper published in the Journal of Physiology Dec, 2017; pre-diabetic mice were fed a calorie unrestricted high sugar, high fat but low-BCAA diet. In spite of the high sugar and high fat the mice experienced improvement in metabolic health.
6. Too much protein can cause dehydration because our kidneys would work overtime to remove the excess nitrogen.

Recommendation:

1. Animal proteins are usually complete sources of protein but not consuming plant-based food in our diet could lead to serious problems as plants are excellent sources of a number of anti-oxidants, micronutrients and fiber. Depending on your age, gender, fitness level, lifestyle, workout schedule and fitness goals your protein requirement would vary. As long as you eat plenty of fruits and vegetables, it is ok to consume dairy, meat and fish as the primary sources of protein. Some of the best sources of protein are Whey and eggs.
2. Even though whole grains, nuts and seeds individually are not complete protein, they are excellent sources of protein. Keep in mind that our body needs only 9 amino acids. When we measure protein in our diet we measure both the essential and non-essential amino acids. Bottom line, the source of protein and the profile of amino acids it contains matters much more than just gobbling down a lot of protein. We basically need ONLY the essential amino acids (that's why they are called essential, our body can make the others from them depending on its requirements). It's ok to have non-essential amino acids in our diet but we don't really need a lot of them.
3. If you are a competitive athlete or a bodybuilder it is ideal to have half the protein coming from animal food and other half from plant food. I understand that it's not always possible especially if you are competing but try to eat as much vegetables and whole grain-based food in your diet as possible.
4. Soy protein is a bit controversial for men since soy contain estrogen mimickers.
5. Document your daily protein intake in your journal.

Reduce your Sodium consumption

The recommended limit for salt, according to American Heart Association is 1500 milligrams per day. However, American adults on an average eat more than 3400 milligrams per day. That's more than double the recommended limit.

Facts:

1. According to Centers for Disease Control (CDC) food bought from retail stores account for around 65% of our daily intake of salt whereas food eaten at restaurants account for 25%. Only 10% of the total daily salt intake comes from home cooking.
2. Highly processed foods or food served in restaurants like breads and rolls, pizza, sandwiches, cold cut and cured meats, soups and burritos and tacos, pack a big sodium punch and should be avoided as much as possible.
3. High blood pressure is one the major causes of death among women in America claiming nearly 200,000 lives every year. Nearly 80 million American adults have high blood pressure. Unfortunately, many food companies and restaurants are tweaking their recipes to cut the sodium by adding other synthetic additives to keep the processed food appealing to us. That's why we would strongly recommend to avoid processed food and try cooking as much of your food at home as possible.
4. Although as hard as it may sound please do not reduce sodium to below 500 milligrams per day. Sodium is essential for proper functioning of nerves and plays an important role in regulating blood pressure.
5. A study conducted in 2006 at University of Helsinki concluded that increased intake of salt produces thirst which in turn leads to excessive intake of sugary beverages. The intake of soda and beverages has led to an exponential increase in diabetes, heart disease and chronic metabolic disorders. Turns out that the sugary beverages themselves contain added salt.
6. Meta-analysis of existing data conducted at John Hopkins in Oct 2016 concluded that sodium has a positive correlation with increased BMI and waist circumference.
7. When blood sodium is too high our kidneys have to work much harder to maintain the electrolyte and fluid balance in our body.

Recommendations:

1. Cook!
2. Eat fresh instead of packaged food.
3. Avoid soda and beverages.
4. If you have to buy processed food, check the label.
5. The best insurance policy against taking excessive sodium is to keep track of your daily sodium intake in your journal.

Meditation

Facts:

1. A study conducted by researchers at Harvard, Yale and MIT found evidence that meditation increased the size of our brain especially the parts of the brain that deal with processing physical input and attention. It was also observed that some part of the gray matter got thicker in elder individuals who had been practicing meditation for over 10 years. Surprisingly, this part of neo cortex shrinks as we get older.
2. Meditation makes us happier. Research suggests that those who practice meditation have a more active pre-frontal cortex. Pre-frontal cortex enhances the flow of logic and constructive thoughts, thereby inducing positive emotions and mitigating the cortisol induced fight and flight response.
3. Researchers at the University of Wisconsin found that those who practice meditation have reduced anxiety and stress since the part of the brain that regulates these emotions becomes less active. It is hypothesized that meditation helps focus on simple everyday moments without distraction and thus the mind remains calm even in stressful situations. Stress due to uncertain future, financial problems, career changes, family and social stresses are substantially mitigated in those who practice meditation consistently.
4. Mindfulness meditation has been shown to sharpen memory. Some of the other documented benefits of meditation are a) Decrease in pain perception b) reduction in heart attack risk and lowering of blood pressure c) improved digestion d) enhanced creativity e) helps in staying focused and cultivating habits that can lead to weight loss (American Psychology Association, Emotion, 2007).
5. Finally, meditation enhances our quality of sleep. 33% of Americans suffer from sleep deprivation. A study which appeared in Harvard's health blog confirms that a relaxation response is triggered almost immediately by meditation.

Recommendations:

1. Start with 10 mins of meditation every day and gradually increase the duration.
2. There are several ways of doing meditation but I would recommend, in the beginning you start by sitting on a chair and start with mindfulness meditation. In mindfulness meditation the meditator focuses on his/her own breathing as a way of warding off distraction. If you get distracted try to bring your attention back to breathing. You may be distracted a lot initially but as you practice to focus on a particular object or activity you'll begin to notice the benefits of meditation.
3. If you don't notice the benefits right away, I would recommend not to give up and give meditation at least 30 days before giving up.

Read nutrition labels

Most of the produce in the supermarket in its natural or least processed form doesn't have a nutrition label attached to it. And even some like eggs, dairy, milk or fish may have a label in their unprocessed or lightly processed form, they are way superior as nutritionally dense and healthy food than highly processed, sugary, calorically dense and nutritionally devoid food.

Recommendations:

1. Check out the number of servings on the label. You may be surprised to find that something like a half pound banana bread might look appealing based on 1 serving size (approximately 140 calories) but you might change your mind once you realize that it contains over 5 servings.
2. Keep an eye on the fiber content of the food you buy. As discussed in the section on fiber, synthetic fiber is added to processed food to make them look appealing to people who are health conscious. And although some fiber is better than no fiber, the processed food containing synthetic fiber often contains a lot of unwanted ingredients with esoteric chemical names and a significant amount of sugar per serving. Foods such as black beans, nuts and lentils naturally have high dietary fiber.
3. As discussed in the section on protein, high protein in our diets increases the overall thermic effect of food. Therefore, proteins along with fiber make us feel fuller. However too much protein without enough fiber can cause serious metabolic and lower digestive tract problems in future.
4. Please keep an eye on sugar. Food with too much added sugar per serving MUST be avoided. As a rule of thumb, you should limit the added sugar content from all foods to under 25 grams per day and under no circumstances it should exceed over 50 grams.
5. As discussed in the section on salts, keep an eye on the sodium content of processed food. Often canned food, chips, snacks have very high sodium content. Try to limit your daily salt intake to around 1500 milligrams per day and under no circumstances it should exceed over 2300 milligrams per day.
6. Highly processed food often has a very large list of ingredients, a lot of those are chemicals we haven't heard of. As a general rule, processed food with over 10 ingredients must be avoided as the number of ingredients is directly proportional to the amount of physical and chemical treatment the food has undergone before being packaged. Foods with relatively smaller number of ingredients are therefore better. Another thing to keep in mind while going through the list of ingredients is the order in which they've been listed. Usually the ingredients which are the biggest constituent of the product are listed at the top and those that are added in trace amounts are usually at the bottom. Also look for sugar substitutes present in the ingredient list and finally if the word "partially hydrogenated" appears on the list it is better to avoid such products since they may contain trans-fats.
7. Don't be fooled by added micronutrients to processed food or beverages. Often the processing devoids the food of essential micronutrients and they are artificially added to make them look healthy.

Have diversity in diet

From evolutionary standpoint the species that relied on a diverse range of food sources to fuel its needs was more likely to survive during adversity. Therefore, diversity in food has a positive correlation with stability. At the individual level that also implies that the individual has more access to not only macronutrients but a wide variety of sources to drive essential micronutrients.

Facts:

1. According to the Triage Theory, proposed by Dr. Bruce Anmes, when essential macronutrient, vitamins and minerals are inadequate, the bodily systems that are essential to sustain life take precedence over others. However, if the deficiency continues over a long period of time it could lead to chronic disorders. In the current environment of highly processed food, natural foods that contain plenty of essential micronutrients and anti-oxidants have been left aside, leading to major deficiencies and chronic disorders. Invariably, we see certain diets where it is advised that entire macronutrient categories should be removed from our diet to achieve "quick" weight loss goals. And although these diets may have medical short term benefits they are not advisable over a long period of time. In the past we have branded one group of macronutrients (fats) as bad, tried to replace them with sugar from our diet and are now enduring the consequences. Thus, before we eliminate any other dietary macronutrient from our diet and go from one extreme to another we should consider the effects of the processed food industry on our diet and on our mindsets.
2. As discussed in the section on fiber, gut microbiome flourish when we have a diversity in our diets. That is, diversity in diet leads to a diversity in our microbiome flora. The more diverse the microbiome, the better the immune system, stronger the anti-inflammatory response leading to reduction in the number of individuals suffering from metabolic disorders. Since our microbiome depends on our diet, someone who's heavily dependent on processed food and sweetened beverages would have very different and significantly less diverse microbiome flora in their gut than someone who espouses minimally processed food.
3. Research suggest that children under the age of 12 months who are given the same food over and over again are more prone to food intolerance and allergic reactions.
4. A diverse plant-based diet has also been shown to reduce lipid peroxidation and DNA oxidation which is a common cause of several diseases. It has been observed that consuming multi-colored fruit and vegetable diet would provide wide variety of antioxidants to the body thereby significantly reducing oxidative stress.

Recommendation:

1. Diversity can be useful but please don't stretch it too far. Eating around 10 to 12 different fruits and vegetables every week is diverse enough for a healthy living. To make things interesting you may try adding or removing a few every other week for a change. Please do not go overboard with it. Recent research indicates that eating food just for the sake of diversity can lead to unnecessary food consumption.

Carbohydrates and Fats

Facts:

1. Recently carbohydrates as a group have been branded as the "bad" component of our diet. We are being told over and over again that we should cut back on our intake of carbohydrates. (Just like we were told 30 years ago that we should cut back our intake of dietary fats.). It is advertised that carbohydrates are responsible for our current obesity and metabolic predicament. Therefore, several diets like paleo diet and ketogenic diets have become popular since they advocate reduction or even removal of carbohydrates from our diets. However past experience has taught us that going to extremes with macronutrients could lead to disastrous consequences.
2. The problem with sugar, as we have already discussed, is that in its processed form, it is rapidly absorbed in the small intestine leading to a spike in blood glucose and insulin levels. However, fruits such as mangoes, apples, sugarcane contain not only sugar but a lot of fiber and micronutrients as well. When we consume these fruits, the fiber slows the absorption of sugar and thus there is a slow rise in blood glucose and insulin levels. This is much healthier than the rapid rise in insulin when sugar is taken directly or when eat processed food bloated with added sugar. These kind of foods like nuts, seeds, fruits and vegetables are called low glycemic index food. The rate at which glucose is discharged in the blood stream is called the glycemic index of that food. Whole grains, seeds, nuts and quinoa cause a slower release of glucose in the blood stream and therefore the insulin response is milder.
3. Almost all processed food with added sugar are high glycemic index food. High glycemic index food are less satiating, due to lack of fiber and protein, and could result in overeating and/or quicker return of hunger.
4. In the late 1970's fats were labeled as the unhealthy component of our diet and we were advised to reduce our fat consumption. Fat free and low-fat food products became popular and the food industry replaced fat in the food with sugar. Reduction or even altogether elimination of fats caused health problems since fat a)support the absorption of vitamins, b)are required to keep heart and blood vessels healthy, c)help brain development and function, d)help in building structural components of cells and e)provide an additional source of energy.
5. There are two types of fats: unsaturated fats and saturated fats. Saturated fats are solid at room temperature and primarily comprise of animal fats. Unsaturated fats on the other hand are liquid at room temperature. There is a subtype of unsaturated fatty acids called Omega-3's. Omega-3's are the only fatty acids that are essential of us since the human body cannot produce them.
6. Fats found in seeds, nuts and avocados are unsaturated fats.
7. When unsaturated fats are hydrogenated they could produce trans-fats. Trans-fats are found in oils that are often used more than once, cooled and used again. Trans-fats are bad for health and if consumed could severely compromise our heart health.

Recommendation:

1. Avoid foods with high glycemic index. Eat unsaturated fats, reduce the consumption of saturated fats and avoid trans fats altogether.

Sleep

Facts:

1. During our sleep our body recharges and repairs itself. Various neurotransmitters and hormones are released which heal and repair our damaged systems. Our immune system supplemented by our microbiome plays a key role in repair. Therefore at least 7 hours of sleep is necessary for maintaining good health.
2. Research suggests that Americans on an average sleep an hour less than what they used to in 1940.
3. Research also suggests that if while in sleep a deep sleep simulating sound is played at the same burst frequency as people's brain wave then people tend to go to "deep sleep" faster and they stay in deep sleep longer.
4. Based on meta-analysis conducted by Public Health England it was concluded that there is growing empirical and experimental evidence that health problems like obesity, heart disease, diabetes and other metabolic disorders could be exacerbated or fueled by lack of sleep. Lack of sleep has been attributed to mental health, poor performance on tests, Alzheimer and memory disorders.
5. Sleep Apnea is one of the side effects of obesity and affects the quality of sleep. It's like a vicious cycle where lack of sleep causes fatigue, slow reaction time, neurotransmitter imbalance, increase in cortisol level and hormonal imbalance thereby resulting in an increase in weight. However, increase in weight causes sleep apnea and sleep apnea worsens the quality of sleep thereby increasing the weight further.
6. Turns out that the reverse is also true. Researchers found that oversleeping can also have serious consequences on our health. People who slept more than 10 hours a day had disrupted sleep cycles, hormonal imbalance, impaired glucose tolerance and gained weight. Thus, people who overslept were likely to become obese or are already obese.

Recommendations:

1. Try to sleep for at least 7 hours a day. 7 to 9 hours of sleep a day is considered healthy.
2. If you are wide awake late at night and cannot go to sleep, the following may help: a) lower the thermostat b) take a shower before going to bed c) Immerse your face in very cold water for 30 seconds d) don't consume caffeine in the evening e) meditate f) work out regularly g) give up sugary and processed food.

Drink Water

Humans cannot survive for more than 3 days without water although we can survive without food for as much as 3 weeks.

Facts:

1. The enzymatic action and hormonal responses are reduced substantially due to dehydration thereby slowing down our response time, making us feel tired and fatigued.
2. Our blood is over 90% water when fully hydrated. When dehydrated however, our blood gets thicker leading to increased resistance to blood flow and thereby resulting in high blood pressure.
3. Our skin removes toxins from our body via sweating. However, when water is low the toxins get stuck under the skin leading to dermatitis, wrinkling, discoloration and even infection. Chronic dehydration is also responsible for wrinkled and withered skin thus leading to premature aging.
4. Research suggest that a person who is dehydrated would not lose fat since most of the toxins that are not eliminated due to dehydration are put aside in fat cells. The body cannot safely remove toxins unless properly hydrated. Therefore, proper hydration is directly related to fat loss.
5. Research suggest that preloading water before a meal could reduce appetite thus reducing the number of calories you will consume.
6. Drinking cold water can speed up metabolism but will not affect the calories burnt in any significant way.
7. Scientists estimated that by just increasing the water consumption to 1.5 liters a day (8 cups of 8 oz) could lead to an estimated weight loss of upto five pounds in one year, assuming all other variables remain unchanged.

Recommendation:

1. Drink at least 2 cups of water before every meal and try to drink 1.5 to 2 liters of water a day.

Avoid antibiotics as much as possible

United States has less than 5% of the world population and consumes nearly 50% of the total antibiotics manufactured in the world. The misuse of antibiotics is rampant. More than 90% of physicians prescribe antibiotics to their patients even when it is not necessary.

Facts:

1. Antibiotics can significantly change our gut flora to such an extent that some of the species can be entirely wiped out. Diversity in our gut microbiome is an indicator of good digestive health. Antibiotics as the name suggest kills the bacteria including those that have a synergistic relationship with us. Research suggests that if newborns are given doses of antibiotics before the age of one year their immune system may get seriously compromised for life. It was further observed that a lot of patients suffering from chronic health disorders especially metabolic, digestive, allergic and immune problems were given lots of antibiotics as kids for minor infections, more than 50% of which don't require antibiotics.
2. Even if you've been given antibiotics in the past, your gut will repair itself if you stop using unnecessary antibiotics (or use them only when absolutely necessary).

Recommendations:

1. If you are sick, you may require antibiotics, but before you are prescribed, ask your doctor about the effects of antibiotics on your immune system and digestive system. And based on the symptoms you are suffering from, is it necessary to use antibiotics. Antibiotics are going to have side effects and they are going to change the profile of your gut microbiome if used for a long time or at a heavy dose.
2. Eat antibiotic free food. Almost 3/4th of the antibiotics used in United States is used on farm animals. These antibiotics eventually enter our system as we consume dairy, poultry and meat. However, they not only inflict damage to our immune system and microbiome they also bring us antibiotic resistant bacteria also called "Super bugs". Super bugs in the past have been traced directly to chicken and meat.

What is NNT ?

Number needed to treat (NNT) is defined as the number of patients required to treat with a drug or medical procedure, to prevent one bad outcome or the number of patients that need to be treated for one to experience benefit or removal of symptoms. That means if the NNT for say a diabetes medication is 25 then you have to treat 25 people to prevent diabetes in 1.

Facts:

1. The treatment of most metabolic diseases like type 2 diabetes, heart diseases, hypertension and other serious ailments often have medications and medical procedures with high NNT. In Pharmacoeconomics NNT is a significant factor. Health insurers are averse to providing coverage for medications with high NNT.
2. Although NNT is an important number, it should be taken with a grain of salt. For example, several clinical trials require administration of drug or medical procedure for several months if not years and finding, for how many patients the drug has prevented a bad outcome or benefited them quantitatively is a difficult task which requires a lot of probabilistic and statistical analysis.
3. Almost all drugs used to treat chronic metabolic disorders have side effects. In fact, the probability of side effects of some drugs is higher than that of NNT. That means if you happen to take those drugs with high NNT and high side effects, you are more likely to get side effects than benefits.
4. It is hard to compare NNT clinical trials because they are dependent on the duration of the clinical trial. Also, for most drugs it is hard to find significant number of studies for an accurate NNT. That being said, it is still worth knowing the NNT of a medication.
5. Example: If the mortality rate from type-2 diabetes in 5 years without the intervention of a medication (say Drug -ABC1) is 25% and after the intervention of the drug is 20%. Then the NNT for the drug ABC1 is:

$$1/(\text{Absolute Risk Reduction}) = 1/(0.25 - 0.20) = 1/0.05 = 20.$$

Do research before going on Fad diets

There are hundreds of so called get slim quick diets. Hardly any of them are backed up by clinical trials and scientific evidences. Yet hundreds of millions of people follow these diets and many actually do lose weight on them, however more than 98% of them regain the lost weight within 3 years.

Facts:

1. There are several diets that encourage people to adapt unorthodox guidelines and rules to lose weight quickly. For example, chew food 32 times, eat only cabbage, low carb diet, juice diet, grapefruit diet, 5-byte diets, carnivore diet. Some of them can not only cause serious nutritional deficiency and lower your metabolism but could be outright dangerous and could exacerbate underlying medical conditions if present.
2. However, there are some diets that have helped people lose weight like Atkins diet, paleo diet, ketogenic diet, vegan diet, 5:2 diet (5:2 diet comes under the broader umbrella of intermittent fasting, which is not exactly a "diet" per se and has shown results similar to calorie restriction in clinical trials).
3. Ketogenic diet is a high fat low, low carb diet. Research suggests that ketogenic diet could be very useful for patients suffering from seizures. However, there is limited data to suggest ketogenic diets efficacy in the treatment for Alzheimer's disease, ALS, autism and cancer. Some trials on cancer research provided evidence that ketogenic diet may be useful in treating certain cancers whereas other trials found no such correlation. Research also suggests that overweight and obese individuals who followed ketogenic diets have experienced significant weight loss. However, owing to the low fiber content the diet is considered unhealthy and not feasible in the long run without medical supervision. It was further noticed that the weight lost during the diet was regained after the diet.
4. Although eating majority plant-based food has several health benefits, completely giving up on animal food like dairy, poultry, fish and meat may cause nutritional deficiency. People undertake vegan diet for several reasons including but not limited to better health, weight loss, animal rights etc. There have been several studies done that show a positive correlation between vegan diet and a reduction in the occurrence of certain types of cancer. Nonetheless, as discussed in the section on proteins, several animal products are complete protein and unlike plant protein, are very high in protein content. Eliminating dairy entails vegan dieters to get adequate sources of calcium. Based on an interesting research there is also evidence that suggests that those who eat unprocessed or lightly processed fruits, vegetables and whole grains complemented by physical exercise have a higher longevity.

Recommendations:

1. Stay away from diets that require you to 1) cut back on calories via unorthodox tactics 2) cut back on calories by removing entire food groups (although there could be exceptions like ketogenic diet and vegan diet) 3) only eat specific foods with prescribed combinations 4) cleanse your body using so called super foods, cleansers etc.
2. Although I won't recommend them, you may try ketogenic diet, intermittent fasting or vegan diet for a short period of time. They have certain benefits in the short term but there are no long-term clinical studies done to support the long-term claims. However, if you follow the guidelines and recommendations in this book you probably won't need to do any diet.
3. Keto food, paleo food, low carb drinks, pre-workout drinks, post-workout drinks, inter-workout drinks are almost always marketing gimmicks. If you do want to try out ketogenic diet or intermittent fasting or vegan diet you don't have to buy overly processed food or drinks to try them out. Please stay away from processed food.